LOW CARB VEGETARIAN MEAL PLAN FOR TYPE 2 DIABETES

Delicious Recipes for Managing Type 2 Diabetes with a Low-Carb Vegetarian Diet

By Mia Bennett

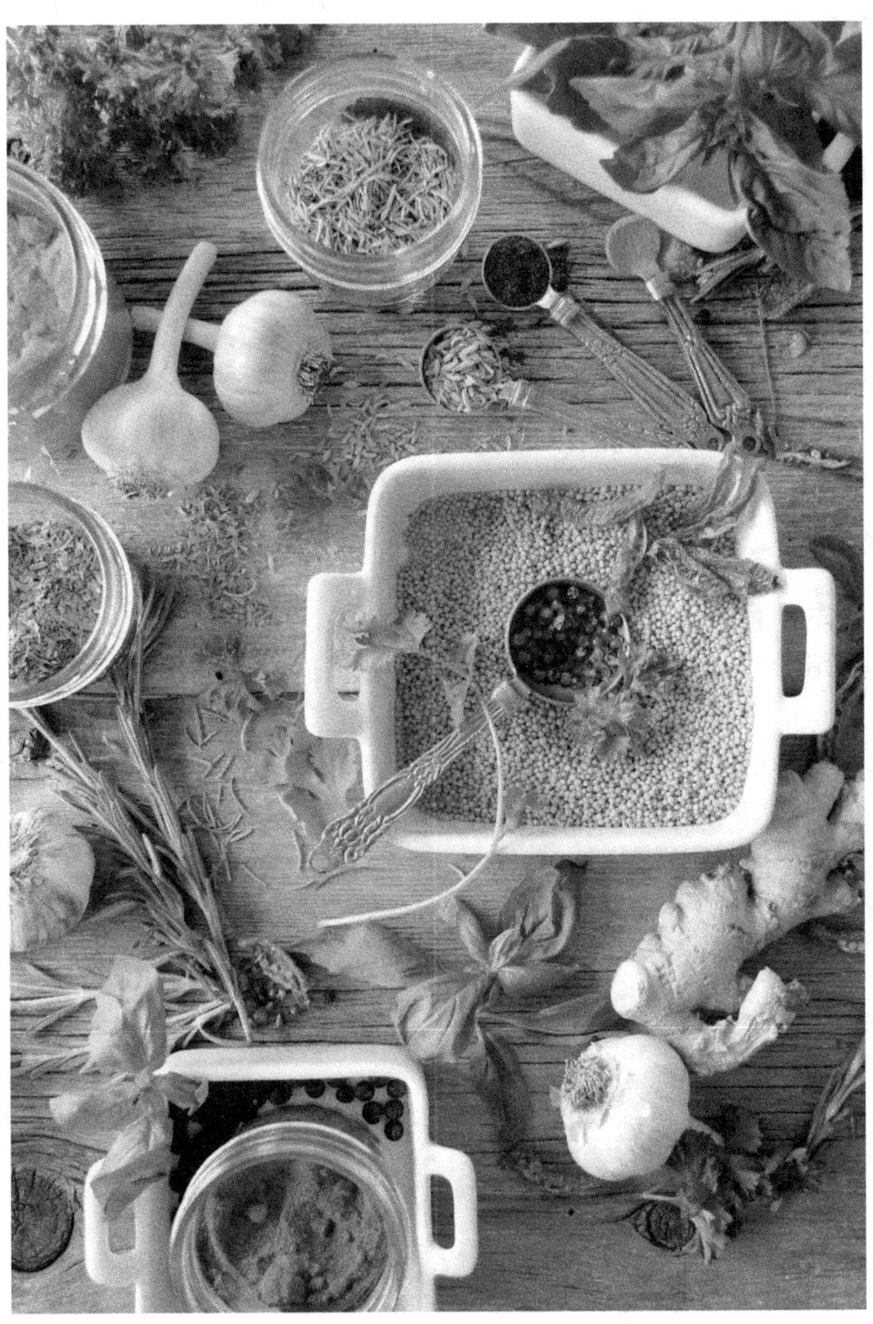

TABLE OF CONTENTS

Chapter 3: Lunch Recipes 39

Chapter 4: Dinner Recipes 57

Chapter 5: Snacks and Appetizers 75

Chapter 6: Desserts 90

Chapter 7: Smoothies 108

INTRODUCTION

I magine your body is a grand orchestra, and blood sugar acts like the conductor. In type 2 diabetes, this conductor struggles to keep the music smooth. Food choices become like instruments - some create sweet harmony, while others cause discord. Here's how to understand the music and create a delicious symphony with a low-carb vegetarian diet.

Type 2 Diabetes: A Body Out of Tune

Our bodies convert food into energy, primarily through sugar (glucose) in the bloodstream. Insulin, a hormone, acts like a key, unlocking cells to absorb this sugar. In type 2 diabetes, either the body doesn't produce enough insulin, or cells become resistant to its effects. This disrupts the flow, leading to high blood sugar levels.

The Low-Carb Vegetarian Advantage: A Lighter Score

Carbohydrates are the main culprit for blood sugar spikes. A low-carb vegetarian diet reduces these spikes by focusing on plant-based proteins, healthy fats, and low-glycemic vegetables. This creates a smoother melody for your blood sugar, promoting better control and overall health.

Benefits of the Low-Carb Vegetarian Symphony

- **Weight Management:** Shedding excess pounds can significantly improve blood sugar control. Plant-based proteins and fiber in this diet keep you feeling fuller for longer, aiding weight management.
- **Improved Heart Health:** This dietary approach is naturally lower in saturated fats and cholesterol, promoting a healthier cardiovascular system.
- **Enhanced Energy Levels:** Stable blood sugar translates to steady energy. No more afternoon slumps or sugar crashes!

Using the Low-Carb Vegetarian Meal Plan

This meal plan provides a roadmap for your dietary symphony. Think of it as a starting point - customize portion sizes and explore recipe variations to suit your taste. Remember, consistency is key!

- **Planning is Paramount**: Dedicate some time each week to plan meals and grocery lists. This reduces the risk of unhealthy choices when hunger strikes.

- **Read Labels Like a Maestro**: Become familiar with carbohydrate content and choose low-glycemic options. There's a world of delicious low-carb veggies waiting to be explored!

- **Embrace Variety:** Don't be afraid to experiment with different vegetarian protein sources like tofu, lentils, and tempeh. Keep your taste buds engaged!

Essential Ingredients and Kitchen Tools

Spice Rack Symphony: Spices add depth and flavor without added sugars or sodium. Explore herbs like basil, oregano, and cumin to create culinary masterpieces.

- **Food Processor Power:** This tool is a time-saver for chopping vegetables, pureeing sauces, and whipping up dips.

- **Non-Stick Savior:** A good non-stick pan allows you to cook with minimal oil, keeping your meals healthy and flavorful.

Embrace the Journey: A Sustainable Performance

Remember, a healthy lifestyle is a marathon, not a sprint. Celebrate your progress, and don't be discouraged by occasional slip-ups. With a low-carb vegetarian diet, you're not just managing diabetes - you're creating a sustainable symphony of health and well-being.

Chapter 1: 30 Day Meal Plan

Week 1

Day 1:

- Breakfast: Spinach and Feta Omelette
- Lunch: Zucchini Noodles with Pesto
- Dinner: Eggplant Lasagna
- Snack: Guacamole with Cucumber Slices
- Dessert: Chocolate Avocado Mousse

Day 2:

- Breakfast: Greek Yogurt with Berries and Nuts
- Lunch: Lentil and Vegetable Soup
- Dinner: Cauliflower Crust Pizza
- Snack: Roasted Chickpeas
- Dessert: Almond Flour Brownies

Day 3:

- Breakfast: Avocado and Tomato Breakfast Salad
- Lunch: Greek Salad with Tofu
- Dinner: Tofu Stir Fry with Peanut Sauce
- Snack: Avocado Deviled Eggs
- Dessert: Berry Cheesecake Cups

Day 4:

- Breakfast: Chia Seed Pudding with Almond Milk
- Lunch: Cauliflower Rice Stir Fry
- Dinner: Zoodles with Alfredo Sauce
- Snack: Spicy Edamame
- Dessert: Coconut Flour Cookies

Day 5:

- Breakfast: Mushroom and Cheese Frittata
- Lunch: Chickpea and Avocado Salad
- Dinner: Spinach and Ricotta Stuffed Peppers
- Snack: Cauliflower Bites with Buffalo Sauce
- Dessert: Keto Chocolate Chip Cookies

Day 6:

- Breakfast: Low Carb Vegan Pancakes
- Lunch: Stuffed Bell Peppers with Quinoa
- Dinner: Grilled Portobello Mushrooms with Garlic Sauce
- Snack: Cheese and Olive Skewers
- Dessert: Lemon Ricotta Cake

Day 7:

- Breakfast: Cauliflower Hash Browns
- Lunch: Spinach and Feta Stuffed Portobellos

- Dinner: Cauliflower and Broccoli Gratin
- Snack: Kale Chips
- Dessert: Chia Seed Pudding with Cocoa

Week 2

Day 8:

- Breakfast: Tofu Scramble with Veggies
- Lunch: Vegan Cobb Salad
- Dinner: Vegan Shepherd's Pie
- Snack: Greek Yogurt Dip with Veggie Sticks
- Dessert: Almond Butter Fat Bombs

Day 9:

- Breakfast: Almond Flour Muffins
- Lunch: Broccoli and Cheddar Soup
- Dinner: Spicy Thai Peanut Noodles
- Snack: Almond Butter Stuffed Celery
- Dessert: Low Carb Tiramisu

Day 10:

- Breakfast: Cottage Cheese with Cinnamon and Flaxseeds
- Lunch: Eggplant Parmesan
- Dinner: Stuffed Zucchini Boats

- Snack: Marinated Artichoke Hearts
- Dessert: Raspberry Almond Tart

Day 11:

- Breakfast: Green Smoothie Bowl
- Lunch: Cucumber and Hummus Wrap
- Dinner: Vegetable and Tofu Kebabs
- Snack: Low Carb Hummus with Bell Pepper Strips
- Dessert: Peanut Butter Chocolate Bars

Day 12:

- Breakfast: Zucchini Breakfast Boats
- Lunch: Roasted Veggie Salad with Tahini Dressing
- Dinner: Low Carb Veggie Burger
- Snack: Mozzarella and Cherry Tomato Skewers
- Dessert: Coconut Macaroons

Day 13:

- Breakfast: Egg Muffins with Veggies
- Lunch: Spaghetti Squash with Marinara
- Dinner: Baked Ratatouille
- Snack: Spinach and Artichoke Dip
- Dessert: Sugar-Free Lemon Bars

Day 14:

- Breakfast: Keto Granola with Coconut Milk
- Lunch: Kale and Brussels Sprout Salad
- Dinner: Chickpea Curry
- Snack: Zucchini Fritters
- Dessert: Chocolate Chia Pudding

Week 3

Day 15:

- Breakfast: Berry Smoothie with Spinach and Protein Powder
- Lunch: Cauliflower Tabbouleh
- Dinner: Creamy Mushroom Stroganoff
- Snack: Caprese Salad Bites
- Dessert: Strawberry Cream Cheese Bites

Day 16:

- Breakfast: Spinach and Feta Omelette
- Lunch: Zucchini Noodles with Pesto
- Dinner: Eggplant Lasagna
- Snack: Guacamole with Cucumber Slices
- Dessert: Chocolate Avocado Mousse

Day 17:

- Breakfast: Greek Yogurt with Berries and Nuts
- Lunch: Lentil and Vegetable Soup
- Dinner: Cauliflower Crust Pizza
- Snack: Roasted Chickpeas
- Dessert: Almond Flour Brownies

Day 18:

- Breakfast: Avocado and Tomato Breakfast Salad
- Lunch: Greek Salad with Tofu
- Dinner: Tofu Stir Fry with Peanut Sauce
- Snack: Avocado Deviled Eggs
- Dessert: Berry Cheesecake Cups

Day 19:

- Breakfast: Chia Seed Pudding with Almond Milk
- Lunch: Cauliflower Rice Stir Fry
- Dinner: Zoodles with Alfredo Sauce
- Snack: Spicy Edamame
- Dessert: Coconut Flour Cookies

Day 20:

- Breakfast: Mushroom and Cheese Frittata
- Lunch: Chickpea and Avocado Salad

- Dinner: Spinach and Ricotta Stuffed Peppers
- Snack: Cauliflower Bites with Buffalo Sauce
- Dessert: Keto Chocolate Chip Cookies

Day 21:

- Breakfast: Low Carb Vegan Pancakes
- Lunch: Stuffed Bell Peppers with Quinoa
- Dinner: Grilled Portobello Mushrooms with Garlic Sauce
- Snack: Cheese and Olive Skewers
- Dessert: Lemon Ricotta Cake

Week 4

Day 22:

- Breakfast: Cauliflower Hash Browns
- Lunch: Spinach and Feta Stuffed Portobellos
- Dinner: Cauliflower and Broccoli Gratin
- Snack: Kale Chips
- Dessert: Chia Seed Pudding with Cocoa

Day 23:

- Breakfast: Tofu Scramble with Veggies
- Lunch: Vegan Cobb Salad
- Dinner: Vegan Shepherd's Pie

- Snack: Greek Yogurt Dip with Veggie Sticks
- Dessert: Almond Butter Fat Bombs

Day 24:

- Breakfast: Almond Flour Muffins
- Lunch: Broccoli and Cheddar Soup
- Dinner: Spicy Thai Peanut Noodles
- Snack: Almond Butter Stuffed Celery
- Dessert: Low Carb Tiramisu

Day 25:

- Breakfast: Cottage Cheese with Cinnamon and Flaxseeds
- Lunch: Eggplant Parmesan
- Dinner: Stuffed Zucchini Boats
- Snack: Marinated Artichoke Hearts
- Dessert: Raspberry Almond Tart

Day 26:

- Breakfast: Green Smoothie Bowl
- Lunch: Cucumber and Hummus Wrap
- Dinner: Vegetable and Tofu Kebabs
- Snack: Low Carb Hummus with Bell Pepper Strips
- Dessert: Peanut Butter Chocolate Bars

Day 27:

- Breakfast: Zucchini Breakfast Boats
- Lunch: Roasted Veggie Salad with Tahini Dressing
- Dinner: Low Carb Veggie Burger
- Snack: Mozzarella and Cherry Tomato Skewers
- Dessert: Coconut Macaroons

Day 28:

- Breakfast: Egg Muffins with Veggies
- Lunch: Spaghetti Squash with Marinara
- Dinner: Baked Ratatouille
- Snack: Spinach and Artichoke Dip
- Dessert: Sugar-Free Lemon Bars

Day 29:

- Breakfast: Keto Granola with Coconut Milk
- Lunch: Kale and Brussels Sprout Salad
- Dinner: Chickpea Curry
- Snack: Zucchini Fritters
- Dessert: Chocolate Chia Pudding

Day 30:

- Breakfast: Berry Smoothie with Spinach and Protein Powder
- Lunch: Cauliflower Tabbouleh

- Dinner: Creamy Mushroom Stroganoff

- Snack: Caprese Salad Bites

- Dessert: Strawberry Cream Cheese Bites

Chapter 2: Breakfast Recipes

Starting your day with a nutritious, low-carb vegetarian breakfast is a great way to maintain balanced blood sugar levels and provide sustained energy. Here are fifteen breakfast recipes designed specifically for people managing Type 2 diabetes, packed with proteins, healthy fats, and fiber to keep you full and satisfied.

Spinach and Feta Omelette

Ingredients:

- 3 large eggs
- 1 cup fresh spinach, chopped
- 1/4 cup feta cheese, crumbled
- 1 tbsp olive oil
- Salt and pepper to taste

Instructions:

1. Whisk the eggs in a bowl with salt and pepper.
2. Heat olive oil in a non-stick skillet over medium heat.
3. Add spinach and sauté until wilted.
4. Pour eggs over spinach, cook until edges set.
5. Sprinkle feta over one side, fold omelette in half.
6. Cook until cheese melts, about 2 minutes.

Nutrition Information (per serving):

- Calories: 250
- Protein: 16g
- Carbohydrates: 3g
- Fat: 20g
- Fiber: 1g
- Sugar: 1g
- Portion size: 1 omelette

Greek Yogurt with Berries and Nuts

Ingredients:

- 1 cup plain Greek yogurt
- 1/2 cup mixed berries (blueberries, strawberries, raspberries)
- 2 tbsp mixed nuts (almonds, walnuts)
- 1 tsp honey (optional)

Instructions:

1. Place yogurt in a bowl.
2. Top with berries and nuts.
3. Drizzle with honey if desired.

Nutrition Information (per serving):

- Calories: 220

- Protein: 15g

- Carbohydrates: 15g

- Fat: 10g

- Fiber: 4g

- Sugar: 10g

- Portion size: 1 bowl

Avocado and Tomato Breakfast Salad

Ingredients:

- 1 ripe avocado, diced

- 1 cup cherry tomatoes, halved

- 1/4 red onion, finely chopped

- 1 tbsp olive oil

- 1 tbsp lemon juice

- Salt and pepper to taste

Instructions:

1. Combine avocado, tomatoes, and onion in a bowl.

2. Drizzle with olive oil and lemon juice.

3. Season with salt and pepper, toss gently.

Nutrition Information (per serving):

- Calories: 210

- Protein: 3g
- Carbohydrates: 12g
- Fat: 18g
- Fiber: 8g
- Sugar: 4g
- Portion size: 1 salad

Chia Seed Pudding with Almond Milk

Ingredients:

- 1/4 cup chia seeds
- 1 cup unsweetened almond milk
- 1 tsp vanilla extract
- 1 tbsp low-carb sweetener
- Fresh berries for topping

Instructions:

1. Mix chia seeds, almond milk, vanilla, and sweetener in a bowl.
2. Refrigerate for at least 2 hours or overnight.
3. Stir well and top with fresh berries before serving.

Nutrition Information (per serving):

- Calories: 180

- Protein: 5g

- Carbohydrates: 14g

- Fat: 10g

- Fiber: 11g

- Sugar: 2g

- Portion size: 1 cup

Mushroom and Cheese Frittata

Ingredients:

- 6 large eggs

- 1 cup mushrooms, sliced

- 1/2 cup shredded cheese (cheddar or mozzarella)

- 1/4 cup milk (or almond milk)

- 1 tbsp olive oil

- Salt and pepper to taste

Instructions:

1. Preheat oven to 375°F (190°C).

2. Sauté mushrooms in olive oil until tender.

3. Whisk eggs with milk, salt, and pepper.

4. Combine mushrooms and cheese with egg mixture.

5. Pour into a greased baking dish and bake for 20-25 minutes.

Nutrition Information (per serving):

- Calories: 220
- Protein: 15g
- Carbohydrates: 3g
- Fat: 17g
- Fiber: 1g
- Sugar: 1g
- Portion size: 1 slice (1/6 of the frittata)

Low Carb Vegan Pancakes

Ingredients:

- 1 cup almond flour
- 1 tbsp flaxseed meal
- 1/2 cup almond milk
- 1 tbsp coconut oil, melted
- 1 tsp baking powder
- 1 tsp vanilla extract
- Low-carb sweetener to taste

Instructions:

1. Mix all ingredients in a bowl until smooth.
2. Heat a non-stick skillet over medium heat.
3. Pour batter onto skillet, forming small pancakes.

4. Cook until bubbles form, then flip and cook until golden.

Nutrition Information (per serving):

- Calories: 150
- Protein: 6g
- Carbohydrates: 6g
- Fat: 12g
- Fiber: 3g
- Sugar: 1g
- Portion size: 2-3 pancakes

Cauliflower Hash Browns

Ingredients:

- 2 cups cauliflower rice
- 1 egg
- 1/4 cup shredded cheese
- 2 tbsp almond flour
- Salt and pepper to taste
- 1 tbsp olive oil

Instructions:

1. Mix cauliflower, egg, cheese, almond flour, salt, and pepper.
2. Form into patties.

3. Heat olive oil in a skillet over medium heat.

4. Cook patties until golden and crispy on each side.

Nutrition Information (per serving):

- Calories: 120
- Protein: 6g
- Carbohydrates: 5g
- Fat: 8g
- Fiber: 2g
- Sugar: 2g
- Portion size: 2 hash browns

Tofu Scramble with Veggies

Ingredients:

- 1 block firm tofu, crumbled
- 1/2 bell pepper, diced
- 1/2 onion, diced
- 1 cup spinach
- 1 tbsp nutritional yeast
- 1 tsp turmeric
- 1 tbsp olive oil
- Salt and pepper to taste

Instructions:

1. Heat olive oil in a skillet, sauté onion and bell pepper until tender.
2. Add crumbled tofu, turmeric, nutritional yeast, salt, and pepper.
3. Cook until tofu is heated through.
4. Stir in spinach until wilted.

Nutrition Information (per serving):

- Calories: 180
- Protein: 14g
- Carbohydrates: 8g
- Fat: 12g
- Fiber: 4g
- Sugar: 3g
- Portion size: 1 cup

Almond Flour Muffins

Ingredients:

- 2 cups almond flour
- 1/4 cup coconut flour
- 1/4 cup low-carb sweetener
- 3 large eggs

- 1/4 cup melted coconut oil
- 1/2 tsp baking soda
- 1/2 tsp vanilla extract

Instructions:

1. Preheat oven to 350°F (175°C).
2. Mix all ingredients in a bowl until well combined.
3. Pour batter into muffin tin lined with paper cups.
4. Bake for 20-25 minutes until golden.

Nutrition Information (per serving):

- Calories: 150
- Protein: 6g
- Carbohydrates: 6g
- Fat: 12g
- Fiber: 3g
- Sugar: 2g
- Portion size: 1 muffin

Cottage Cheese with Cinnamon and Flaxseeds

Ingredients:

- 1 cup cottage cheese

- 1 tbsp ground flaxseeds

- 1/2 tsp ground cinnamon

- Low-carb sweetener to taste

Instructions:

1. Combine cottage cheese, flaxseeds, and cinnamon in a bowl.

2. Add sweetener to taste and mix well.

Nutrition Information (per serving):

- Calories: 180

- Protein: 14g

- Carbohydrates: 8g

- Fat: 10g

- Fiber: 3g

- Sugar: 4g

- Portion size: 1 cup

Green Smoothie Bowl

Ingredients:

- 1 cup spinach

- 1/2 avocado

- 1/2 cup unsweetened almond milk

- 1 tbsp chia seeds

- 1/4 cup mixed berries for topping

Instructions:

1. Blend spinach, avocado, and almond milk until smooth.
2. Pour into a bowl, top with chia seeds and berries.

Nutrition Information (per serving):

- Calories: 220
- Protein: 5g
- Carbohydrates: 14g
- Fat: 17g
- Fiber: 9g
- Sugar: 4g
- Portion size: 1 bowl

Zucchini Breakfast Boats

Ingredients:

- 2 large zucchinis, halved and scooped out
- 4 eggs
- 1/2 cup diced tomatoes
- 1/4 cup shredded cheese
- Salt and pepper to taste

Instructions:

1. Preheat oven to 375°F (190°C).

2. Place zucchini halves in a baking dish.

3. Crack an egg into each zucchini half.

4. Top with tomatoes and cheese.

5. Bake for 20-25 minutes until eggs are set.

Nutrition Information (per serving):

- Calories: 180

- Protein: 12g

- Carbohydrates: 6g

- Fat: 12g

- Fiber: 2g

- Sugar: 4g

- Portion size: 2 halves

Egg Muffins with Veggies

Ingredients:

- 6 large eggs

- 1/2 cup diced bell pepper

- 1/2 cup chopped spinach

- 1/4 cup shredded cheese

- Salt and pepper to taste

Instructions:

1. Preheat oven to 350°F (175°C).
2. Whisk eggs with salt and pepper.
3. Add bell pepper, spinach, and cheese.
4. Pour mixture into greased muffin tin.
5. Bake for 15-20 minutes until set.

Nutrition Information (per serving):

- Calories: 120
- Protein: 8g
- Carbohydrates: 2g
- Fat: 8g
- Fiber: 1g
- Sugar: 1g
- Portion size: 2 muffins

Keto Granola with Coconut Milk

Ingredients:

- 1 cup mixed nuts (almonds, pecans, walnuts)
- 1/2 cup unsweetened coconut flakes
- 1/4 cup pumpkin seeds
- 1/4 cup melted coconut oil
- 1 tsp cinnamon

- Low-carb sweetener to taste

- 1/2 cup unsweetened coconut milk

Instructions:

1. Preheat oven to 300°F (150°C).

2. Mix nuts, coconut flakes, pumpkin seeds, coconut oil, cinnamon, and sweetener.

3. Spread on a baking sheet and bake for 20 minutes, stirring halfway.

4. Serve with coconut milk.

Nutrition Information (per serving):

- Calories: 250

- Protein: 5g

- Carbohydrates: 8g

- Fat: 22g

- Fiber: 5g

- Sugar: 2g

- Portion size: 1/2 cup granola with 1/2 cup coconut milk

Berry Smoothie with Spinach and Protein Powder

Ingredients:

- 1/2 cup mixed berries (blueberries, raspberries, strawberries)
- 1 cup spinach
- 1 scoop protein powder
- 1 cup unsweetened almond milk
- 1 tbsp chia seeds

Instructions:

1. Blend all ingredients until smooth.
2. Pour into a glass and serve immediately.

Nutrition Information (per serving):

- Calories: 200
- Protein: 20g
- Carbohydrates: 14g
- Fat: 8g
- Fiber: 7g
- Sugar: 6g
- Portion size: 1 smoothie

Chapter 3: Lunch Recipes

Creating a diverse and nutritious lunch is essential for maintaining energy levels and keeping blood sugar stable throughout the day, especially for those managing Type 2 diabetes. The following 15 lunch recipes are designed to be low in carbs while being rich in flavor and nutrients.

Zucchini Noodles with Pesto

Ingredients:

- 2 large zucchinis, spiralized
- 1 cup fresh basil leaves
- 1/4 cup pine nuts
- 1/4 cup grated Parmesan cheese
- 2 garlic cloves
- 1/4 cup olive oil
- Salt and pepper to taste

Instructions:

1. Blend basil, pine nuts, Parmesan, garlic, and olive oil until smooth.
2. Toss zucchini noodles with pesto sauce.
3. Season with salt and pepper.

Nutrition Information (per serving):

- Calories: 200
- Protein: 6g
- Carbohydrates: 8g
- Fat: 17g
- Fiber: 2g
- Sugar: 4g
- Portion size: 1 bowl

Lentil and Vegetable Soup

Ingredients:

- 1 cup lentils
- 1 carrot, diced
- 1 celery stalk, diced
- 1 onion, chopped
- 2 garlic cloves, minced
- 4 cups vegetable broth
- 1 tsp cumin
- 1 tsp paprika
- Salt and pepper to taste

Instructions:

1. Sauté onion, garlic, carrot, and celery in a pot until soft.

2. Add lentils, broth, cumin, and paprika.

3. Simmer for 30 minutes until lentils are tender.

4. Season with salt and pepper.

Nutrition Information (per serving):

- Calories: 180

- Protein: 12g

- Carbohydrates: 30g

- Fat: 2g

- Fiber: 12g

- Sugar: 5g

- Portion size: 1 cup

Greek Salad with Tofu

Ingredients:

- 1 block firm tofu, cubed

- 1 cucumber, diced

- 1 bell pepper, diced

- 1/2 red onion, sliced

- 1/2 cup Kalamata olives

- 1 cup cherry tomatoes, halved

- 1/4 cup feta cheese, crumbled

- 2 tbsp olive oil

- 1 tbsp red wine vinegar
- 1 tsp dried oregano
- Salt and pepper to taste

Instructions:

1. Toss tofu, cucumber, bell pepper, onion, olives, and tomatoes in a bowl.
2. Drizzle with olive oil, vinegar, and sprinkle with oregano.
3. Top with feta cheese and season with salt and pepper.

Nutrition Information (per serving):

- Calories: 250
- Protein: 12g
- Carbohydrates: 10g
- Fat: 18g
- Fiber: 4g
- Sugar: 4g
- Portion size: 1 bowl

Cauliflower Rice Stir Fry

Ingredients:

- 1 head cauliflower, riced
- 1 cup mixed vegetables (carrots, peas, bell peppers)

- 2 garlic cloves, minced
- 2 tbsp soy sauce
- 1 tbsp olive oil
- 1 tsp sesame oil
- 2 green onions, chopped

Instructions:

1. Heat olive oil in a pan and sauté garlic.
2. Add mixed vegetables and cook until tender.
3. Stir in cauliflower rice and soy sauce, cook for 5 minutes.
4. Drizzle with sesame oil and top with green onions.

Nutrition Information (per serving):

- Calories: 150
- Protein: 5g
- Carbohydrates: 12g
- Fat: 10g
- Fiber: 5g
- Sugar: 4g
- Portion size: 1 bowl

Chickpea and Avocado Salad

Ingredients:

- 1 can chickpeas, drained and rinsed
- 1 avocado, diced
- 1 cucumber, diced
- 1/2 red onion, chopped
- 1 tbsp lemon juice
- 2 tbsp olive oil
- Salt and pepper to taste

Instructions:

1. Combine chickpeas, avocado, cucumber, and onion in a bowl.
2. Drizzle with lemon juice and olive oil.
3. Season with salt and pepper.

Nutrition Information (per serving):

- Calories: 280
- Protein: 8g
- Carbohydrates: 24g
- Fat: 18g
- Fiber: 10g
- Sugar: 4g
- Portion size: 1 bowl

Stuffed Bell Peppers with Quinoa

Ingredients:

- 4 bell peppers, tops removed and seeds cleaned
- 1 cup cooked quinoa
- 1 can black beans, drained and rinsed
- 1 cup corn kernels
- 1/2 cup salsa
- 1 tsp cumin
- 1/2 cup shredded cheese

Instructions:

1. Preheat oven to 375°F.
2. Mix quinoa, beans, corn, salsa, and cumin in a bowl.
3. Stuff peppers with the mixture and place in a baking dish.
4. Sprinkle cheese on top and bake for 25 minutes.

Nutrition Information (per serving):

- Calories: 300
- Protein: 12g
- Carbohydrates: 45g
- Fat: 8g
- Fiber: 12g
- Sugar: 10g
- Portion size: 1 stuffed pepper

Spinach and Feta Stuffed Portobellos

Ingredients:

- 4 large portobello mushrooms
- 1 cup spinach, chopped
- 1/2 cup feta cheese, crumbled
- 1 garlic clove, minced
- 2 tbsp olive oil
- Salt and pepper to taste

Instructions:

1. Preheat oven to 375°F.
2. Remove stems from mushrooms and brush caps with olive oil.
3. Sauté spinach and garlic until wilted.
4. Mix in feta cheese and stuff the mixture into mushroom caps.
5. Bake for 20 minutes.

Nutrition Information (per serving):

- Calories: 200
- Protein: 8g
- Carbohydrates: 10g
- Fat: 16g
- Fiber: 4g
- Sugar: 3g

- Portion size: 1 mushroom cap

Vegan Cobb Salad

Ingredients:

- 1 head romaine lettuce, chopped
- 1 avocado, sliced
- 1 cup cherry tomatoes, halved
- 1/2 cup corn kernels
- 1/2 cup black beans, drained and rinsed
- 1/4 cup red onion, chopped
- 1/4 cup vegan bacon bits
- 2 tbsp olive oil
- 1 tbsp balsamic vinegar
- Salt and pepper to taste

Instructions:

1. Toss lettuce, avocado, tomatoes, corn, beans, onion, and bacon bits in a bowl.
2. Drizzle with olive oil and balsamic vinegar.
3. Season with salt and pepper.

Nutrition Information (per serving):

- Calories: 300

- Protein: 8g

- Carbohydrates: 26g

- Fat: 20g

- Fiber: 10g

- Sugar: 6g

- Portion size: 1 bowl

Broccoli and Cheddar Soup

Ingredients:

- 2 cups broccoli florets

- 1 carrot, diced

- 1 celery stalk, diced

- 1 onion, chopped

- 2 cups vegetable broth

- 1 cup shredded cheddar cheese

- 1 cup almond milk

- 2 tbsp olive oil

- Salt and pepper to taste

Instructions:

1. Sauté onion, carrot, and celery in olive oil until soft.

2. Add broccoli and vegetable broth, simmer for 10 minutes.

3. Blend until smooth, then stir in cheese and almond milk.

4. Season with salt and pepper.

Nutrition Information (per serving):

- Calories: 250
- Protein: 10g
- Carbohydrates: 18g
- Fat: 18g
- Fiber: 4g
- Sugar: 6g
- Portion size: 1 cup

Eggplant Parmesan

Ingredients:

- 1 large eggplant, sliced into rounds
- 1 cup marinara sauce
- 1 cup shredded mozzarella cheese
- 1/4 cup grated Parmesan cheese
- 1/4 cup almond flour
- 1 egg, beaten
- 2 tbsp olive oil
- Salt and pepper to taste

Instructions:

1. Preheat oven to 375°F.

2. Dip eggplant slices in egg, then coat with almond flour.

3. Fry in olive oil until golden brown.

4. Layer eggplant, marinara sauce, and cheeses in a baking dish.

5. Bake for 25 minutes.

Nutrition Information (per serving):

- Calories: 300

- Protein: 12g

- Carbohydrates: 20g

- Fat: 22g

- Fiber: 6g

- Sugar: 8g

- Portion size: 1 serving

Cucumber and Hummus Wrap

Ingredients:

- 1 large whole wheat tortilla

- 1/2 cup hummus

- 1 cucumber, sliced

- 1/4 cup shredded carrots

- 1/4 cup red bell pepper, sliced
- 1/4 cup spinach leaves

Instructions:

1. Spread hummus on the tortilla.
2. Layer cucumber, carrots, bell pepper, and spinach on top.
3. Roll up the tortilla tightly.

Nutrition Information (per serving):

- Calories: 250
- Protein: 8g
- Carbohydrates: 34g
- Fat: 10g
- Fiber: 8g
- Sugar: 4g
- Portion size: 1 wrap

Roasted Veggie Salad with Tahini Dressing

Ingredients:

- 1 cup cherry tomatoes
- 1 zucchini, sliced
- 1 bell pepper, sliced

- 1 red onion, sliced

- 2 tbsp olive oil

- 2 cups mixed greens

- 2 tbsp tahini

- 1 tbsp lemon juice

- 1 tbsp water

- Salt and pepper to taste

Instructions:

1. Preheat oven to 400°F.

2. Toss tomatoes, zucchini, bell pepper, and onion with olive oil.

3. Roast for 20 minutes.

4. Mix tahini, lemon juice, and water to make the dressing.

5. Combine roasted veggies with mixed greens and drizzle with dressing.

Nutrition Information (per serving):

- Calories: 220

- Protein: 6g

- Carbohydrates: 20g

- Fat: 14g

- Fiber: 6g

- Sugar: 8g

- Portion size: 1 bowl

Spaghetti Squash with Marinara

Ingredients:

- 1 spaghetti squash
- 2 cups marinara sauce
- 1/4 cup grated Parmesan cheese
- 1 tbsp olive oil
- Salt and pepper to taste

Instructions:

1. Preheat oven to 375°F.
2. Cut squash in half, remove seeds, and brush with olive oil.
3. Bake for 40 minutes until tender.
4. Scrape out strands with a fork and toss with marinara sauce.
5. Top with Parmesan cheese.

Nutrition Information (per serving):

- Calories: 200
- Protein: 6g
- Carbohydrates: 30g
- Fat: 8g
- Fiber: 6g

- Sugar: 10g
- Portion size: 1 bowl

Kale and Brussels Sprout Salad

Ingredients:

- 1 cup kale, chopped
- 1 cup Brussels sprouts, shaved
- 1/4 cup dried cranberries
- 1/4 cup sunflower seeds
- 2 tbsp olive oil
- 1 tbsp apple cider vinegar
- Salt and pepper to taste

Instructions:

1. Toss kale and Brussels sprouts in a bowl.
2. Add cranberries and sunflower seeds.
3. Drizzle with olive oil and apple cider vinegar.
4. Season with salt and pepper.

Nutrition Information (per serving):

- Calories: 220
- Protein: 6g
- Carbohydrates: 22g

- Fat: 14g

- Fiber: 6g

- Sugar: 10g

- Portion size: 1 bowl

Cauliflower Tabbouleh

Ingredients:

- 1 head cauliflower, riced

- 1 cucumber, diced

- 1 tomato, diced

- 1/4 cup parsley, chopped

- 1/4 cup mint, chopped

- 1/4 cup lemon juice

- 2 tbsp olive oil

- Salt and pepper to taste

Instructions:

1. Mix cauliflower, cucumber, tomato, parsley, and mint in a bowl.

2. Drizzle with lemon juice and olive oil.

3. Season with salt and pepper.

Nutrition Information (per serving):

- Calories: 150
- Protein: 4g
- Carbohydrates: 16g
- Fat: 8g
- Fiber: 6g
- Sugar: 6g
- Portion size: 1 bowl

Chapter 4: Dinner Recipes

In this chapter, we will explore a variety of delicious and satisfying low carb vegetarian dinner recipes. These meals focus on fresh vegetables, plant-based proteins, and low-carb alternatives to traditional high-carb dishes. Let's dive into these delectable dinner options!

Eggplant Lasagna

Ingredients:

- 2 large eggplants, sliced lengthwise
- 1 cup ricotta cheese
- 1 cup shredded mozzarella cheese
- 1/2 cup grated Parmesan cheese
- 2 cups marinara sauce
- 1 cup spinach leaves
- 2 cloves garlic, minced
- 1 tbsp olive oil
- Salt and pepper to taste

Instructions:

1. Preheat the oven to 375°F (190°C). Brush eggplant slices with olive oil and bake for 20 minutes.

2. In a bowl, mix ricotta cheese, spinach, and garlic.

3. Layer eggplant slices, ricotta mixture, and marinara sauce in a baking dish. Top with mozzarella and Parmesan.

4. Bake for 25-30 minutes until golden and bubbly.

Nutrition Information (per serving):

- Calories: 250
- Protein: 15g
- Carbohydrates: 15g
- Fat: 15g
- Fiber: 5g
- Sugar: 8g
- Portion size: 1 piece

Cauliflower Crust Pizza

Ingredients:

- 1 large cauliflower head, riced
- 1/2 cup shredded mozzarella cheese
- 1/4 cup grated Parmesan cheese
- 1 egg
- 1 tsp Italian seasoning
- 1/2 cup tomato sauce
- 1 cup mixed vegetables (bell peppers, onions, mushrooms)

- 1/2 cup shredded mozzarella cheese

Instructions:

1. Preheat oven to 400°F (200°C). Mix riced cauliflower, cheeses, egg, and seasoning.
2. Press mixture into a pizza shape on a baking sheet. Bake for 15-20 minutes.
3. Spread tomato sauce on crust, top with vegetables and cheese. Bake for another 10 minutes.

Nutrition Information (per serving):

- Calories: 200
- Protein: 12g
- Carbohydrates: 10g
- Fat: 12g
- Fiber: 3g
- Sugar: 4g
- Portion size: 1 slice

Tofu Stir Fry with Peanut Sauce

Ingredients:

- 1 block firm tofu, cubed
- 2 cups mixed vegetables (broccoli, bell peppers, carrots)

- 2 tbsp peanut butter

- 2 tbsp soy sauce

- 1 tbsp rice vinegar

- 1 clove garlic, minced

- 1 tsp ginger, minced

- 1 tbsp olive oil

Instructions:

1. Heat olive oil in a pan and sauté tofu until golden. Remove from pan.

2. Add vegetables to the pan and cook until tender.

3. Mix peanut butter, soy sauce, rice vinegar, garlic, and ginger in a bowl.

4. Return tofu to the pan, pour sauce over, and stir to coat. Cook for 2-3 more minutes.

Nutrition Information (per serving):

- Calories: 220

- Protein: 15g

- Carbohydrates: 10g

- Fat: 15g

- Fiber: 5g

- Sugar: 3g

- Portion size: 1 bowl

Zoodles with Alfredo Sauce

Ingredients:

- 3 zucchinis, spiralized
- 1 cup heavy cream
- 1/2 cup grated Parmesan cheese
- 1 tbsp butter
- 2 cloves garlic, minced
- Salt and pepper to taste

Instructions:

1. In a saucepan, melt butter and sauté garlic until fragrant.
2. Add heavy cream and Parmesan cheese. Cook until the sauce thickens.
3. Toss zoodles in the sauce and cook for 2-3 minutes until tender.

Nutrition Information (per serving):

- Calories: 220
- Protein: 8g
- Carbohydrates: 7g
- Fat: 18g
- Fiber: 2g
- Sugar: 4g
- Portion size: 1 bowl

Spinach and Ricotta Stuffed Peppers

Ingredients:

- 4 bell peppers, halved and seeded
- 1 cup ricotta cheese
- 1 cup spinach, chopped
- 1/2 cup grated mozzarella cheese
- 1/4 cup grated Parmesan cheese
- 1 egg
- Salt and pepper to taste

Instructions:

1. Preheat oven to 375°F (190°C). Mix ricotta, spinach, mozzarella, Parmesan, egg, salt, and pepper.
2. Stuff bell pepper halves with the mixture.
3. Bake for 25-30 minutes until peppers are tender.

Nutrition Information (per serving):

- Calories: 180
- Protein: 10g
- Carbohydrates: 10g
- Fat: 12g
- Fiber: 3g
- Sugar: 5g
- Portion size: 1 stuffed pepper

Grilled Portobello Mushrooms with Garlic Sauce

Ingredients:

- 4 large Portobello mushrooms
- 1/4 cup olive oil
- 3 cloves garlic, minced
- 1 tbsp balsamic vinegar
- Salt and pepper to taste

Instructions:

1. Preheat grill to medium heat. Mix olive oil, garlic, vinegar, salt, and pepper.
2. Brush mushrooms with the mixture.
3. Grill mushrooms for 5-7 minutes per side until tender.

Nutrition Information (per serving):

- Calories: 150
- Protein: 4g
- Carbohydrates: 8g
- Fat: 12g
- Fiber: 2g
- Sugar: 4g
- Portion size: 1 mushroom

Cauliflower and Broccoli Gratin

Ingredients:

- 1 head cauliflower, cut into florets
- 1 head broccoli, cut into florets
- 1 cup heavy cream
- 1 cup shredded cheddar cheese
- 1/4 cup grated Parmesan cheese
- 1 tbsp butter
- Salt and pepper to taste

Instructions:

1. Preheat oven to 375°F (190°C). Steam cauliflower and broccoli until tender.
2. In a saucepan, melt butter and add cream, cheddar, Parmesan, salt, and pepper. Stir until smooth.
3. Combine vegetables and cheese sauce in a baking dish. Bake for 20 minutes until bubbly.

Nutrition Information (per serving):

- Calories: 220
- Protein: 10g
- Carbohydrates: 8g
- Fat: 18g
- Fiber: 4g

- Sugar: 3g
- Portion size: 1 cup

Vegan Shepherd's Pie

Ingredients:

- 2 cups lentils, cooked
- 1 onion, chopped
- 2 carrots, diced
- 1 cup peas
- 1 cup corn
- 2 cloves garlic, minced
- 2 cups mashed cauliflower
- 1 tbsp olive oil
- Salt and pepper to taste

Instructions:

1. Preheat oven to 375°F (190°C). Sauté onion, carrots, and garlic in olive oil until soft.
2. Add lentils, peas, corn, salt, and pepper. Cook for 5 minutes.
3. Transfer mixture to a baking dish, top with mashed cauliflower.
4. Bake for 20-25 minutes until golden.

Nutrition Information (per serving):

- Calories: 250
- Protein: 12g
- Carbohydrates: 30g
- Fat: 8g
- Fiber: 12g
- Sugar: 6g
- Portion size: 1 cup

Spicy Thai Peanut Noodles

Ingredients:

- 1 package shirataki noodles
- 1/4 cup peanut butter
- 2 tbsp soy sauce
- 1 tbsp sriracha
- 1 tbsp lime juice
- 1 cup mixed vegetables (bell peppers, carrots, snap peas)
- 1 clove garlic, minced

Instructions:

1. Rinse and prepare shirataki noodles according to package instructions.

2. Mix peanut butter, soy sauce, sriracha, lime juice, and garlic in a bowl.

3. Sauté vegetables until tender, add noodles and sauce. Cook for 3-4 minutes.

Nutrition Information (per serving):

- Calories: 180
- Protein: 6g
- Carbohydrates: 10g
- Fat: 12g
- Fiber: 4g
- Sugar: 4g
- Portion size: 1 bowl

Stuffed Zucchini Boats

Ingredients:

- 4 zucchinis, halved and hollowed
- 1 cup quinoa, cooked
- 1 cup black beans, rinsed and drained
- 1 cup corn
- 1/2 cup salsa
- 1/2 cup shredded cheddar cheese
- Salt and pepper to taste

Instructions:

1. Preheat oven to 375°F (190°C). Mix quinoa, beans, corn, salsa, salt, and pepper.
2. Stuff zucchini halves with mixture, top with cheese.
3. Bake for 20-25 minutes until tender.

Nutrition Information (per serving):

- Calories: 200
- Protein: 8g
- Carbohydrates: 25g
- Fat: 8g
- Fiber: 7g
- Sugar: 5g
- Portion size: 1 zucchini half

Vegetable and Tofu Kebabs

Ingredients:

- 1 block firm tofu, cubed
- 1 red bell pepper, chopped
- 1 zucchini, sliced
- 1 red onion, chopped
- 1/4 cup olive oil
- 2 tbsp soy sauce

- 1 tsp garlic powder
- 1 tsp paprika

Instructions:

1. Preheat grill to medium heat. Mix olive oil, soy sauce, garlic powder, and paprika.
2. Thread tofu and vegetables onto skewers, brush with marinade.
3. Grill for 10-12 minutes, turning occasionally.

Nutrition Information (per serving):

- Calories: 180
- Protein: 10g
- Carbohydrates: 8g
- Fat: 12g
- Fiber: 4g
- Sugar: 4g
- Portion size: 2 skewers

Low Carb Veggie Burger

Ingredients:

- 1 cup black beans, mashed
- 1/2 cup grated zucchini

- 1/2 cup grated carrots
- 1/4 cup chopped onions
- 1/4 cup almond flour
- 1 egg
- 1 tsp cumin
- Salt and pepper to taste

Instructions:

1. Preheat oven to 375°F (190°C). Mix all ingredients in a bowl.
2. Form mixture into patties and place on a baking sheet.
3. Bake for 20-25 minutes until firm and golden.

Nutrition Information (per serving):

- Calories: 150
- Protein: 8g
- Carbohydrates: 18g
- Fat: 6g
- Fiber: 6g
- Sugar: 3g
- Portion size: 1 burger

Baked Ratatouille

Ingredients:

- 1 eggplant, sliced
- 1 zucchini, sliced
- 1 yellow squash, sliced
- 1 red bell pepper, sliced
- 1 red onion, sliced
- 2 cups tomato sauce
- 2 cloves garlic, minced
- 1 tbsp olive oil
- Salt and pepper to taste

Instructions:

1. Preheat oven to 375°F (190°C). Layer vegetables in a baking dish.
2. Mix tomato sauce, garlic, olive oil, salt, and pepper. Pour over vegetables.
3. Bake for 30-35 minutes until vegetables are tender.

Nutrition Information (per serving):

- Calories: 180
- Protein: 4g
- Carbohydrates: 20g
- Fat: 10g

- Fiber: 6g
- Sugar: 12g
- Portion size: 1 cup

Chickpea Curry

Ingredients:

- 1 can chickpeas, rinsed and drained
- 1 onion, chopped
- 2 cloves garlic, minced
- 1 can coconut milk
- 2 tbsp curry powder
- 1 cup spinach leaves
- 1 tbsp olive oil
- Salt and pepper to taste

Instructions:

1. Heat olive oil in a pan and sauté onion and garlic until soft.
2. Add chickpeas, curry powder, and coconut milk. Simmer for 10 minutes.
3. Stir in spinach and cook until wilted.

Nutrition Information (per serving):

- Calories: 250

- Protein: 8g

- Carbohydrates: 20g

- Fat: 15g

- Fiber: 6g

- Sugar: 4g

- Portion size: 1 bowl

Creamy Mushroom Stroganoff

Ingredients:

- 2 cups mushrooms, sliced

- 1 onion, chopped

- 2 cloves garlic, minced

- 1 cup vegetable broth

- 1/2 cup sour cream

- 1 tbsp olive oil

- 1 tsp paprika

- Salt and pepper to taste

Instructions:

1. Heat olive oil in a pan and sauté onion, garlic, and mushrooms until soft.

2. Add vegetable broth, paprika, salt, and pepper. Simmer for 5 minutes.

3. Stir in sour cream and cook for another 2-3 minutes until thickened.

Nutrition Information (per serving):

- Calories: 200
- Protein: 6g
- Carbohydrates: 10g
- Fat: 16g
- Fiber: 2g
- Sugar: 4g
- Portion size: 1 cup

Chapter 5: Snacks and Appetizers

Snacking is an integral part of managing hunger and maintaining energy levels throughout the day. For those managing Type 2 diabetes, it's important to choose snacks that are low in carbohydrates but rich in nutrients. The following recipes provide a variety of tasty options that are easy to prepare and perfect for any time of day.

Guacamole with Cucumber Slices

Ingredients:

- 2 ripe avocados
- 1 small red onion, finely chopped
- 1 clove garlic, minced
- 1 lime, juiced
- 1 small tomato, diced
- Salt and pepper to taste
- 1 cucumber, sliced into rounds

Instructions:

1. In a bowl, mash the avocados until smooth.
2. Stir in the red onion, garlic, lime juice, and tomato.
3. Season with salt and pepper.

4. Serve with cucumber slices.

Nutrition Information (per serving, serves 4):

- Calories: 180
- Protein: 2g
- Carbohydrates: 10g
- Fat: 15g
- Fiber: 7g
- Sugar: 2g
- Portion Size: 1/4 cup guacamole with 10 cucumber slices

Roasted Chickpeas

Ingredients:

- 1 can chickpeas, drained and rinsed
- 1 tbsp olive oil
- 1 tsp smoked paprika
- 1/2 tsp garlic powder
- 1/2 tsp salt

Instructions:

1. Preheat oven to 400°F (200°C).
2. Toss chickpeas with olive oil and spices.

3. Spread on a baking sheet and roast for 25-30 minutes, shaking the pan halfway through.

Nutrition Information (per serving, serves 4):

- Calories: 120
- Protein: 5g
- Carbohydrates: 17g
- Fat: 4g
- Fiber: 5g
- Sugar: 0g
- Portion Size: 1/2 cup

Avocado Deviled Eggs

Ingredients:

- 6 hard-boiled eggs, peeled and halved
- 1 ripe avocado
- 1 tsp lemon juice
- 1 tsp Dijon mustard
- Salt and pepper to taste
- Paprika for garnish

Instructions:

1. Remove yolks from eggs and place in a bowl.

2. Add avocado, lemon juice, and mustard. Mash until smooth.

3. Season with salt and pepper.

4. Spoon mixture back into egg whites and sprinkle with paprika.

Nutrition Information (per serving, serves 6):

- Calories: 80
- Protein: 6g
- Carbohydrates: 2g
- Fat: 6g
- Fiber: 1g
- Sugar: 0g
- Portion Size: 1 egg half

Spicy Edamame

Ingredients:

- 2 cups frozen edamame in pods
- 1 tbsp soy sauce
- 1 tsp sesame oil
- 1/2 tsp red pepper flakes

Instructions:

1. Cook edamame according to package instructions.

2. Toss cooked edamame with soy sauce, sesame oil, and red pepper flakes.

Nutrition Information (per serving, serves 4):

- Calories: 120
- Protein: 9g
- Carbohydrates: 10g
- Fat: 6g
- Fiber: 4g
- Sugar: 1g
- Portion Size: 1/2 cup

Cauliflower Bites with Buffalo Sauce

Ingredients:

- 1 small head cauliflower, cut into florets
- 1/4 cup hot sauce
- 2 tbsp melted butter
- 1/2 tsp garlic powder

Instructions:

1. Preheat oven to 450°F (230°C).
2. Toss cauliflower with hot sauce, melted butter, and garlic powder.

3. Spread on a baking sheet and bake for 20 minutes, until tender and slightly crispy.

Nutrition Information (per serving, serves 4):

- Calories: 60
- Protein: 2g
- Carbohydrates: 7g
- Fat: 3g
- Fiber: 3g
- Sugar: 2g
- Portion Size: 1 cup

Cheese and Olive Skewers

Ingredients:

- 1 cup mozzarella balls
- 1 cup mixed olives
- Fresh basil leaves
- Toothpicks or small skewers

Instructions:

1. Thread mozzarella, olives, and basil onto skewers.

Nutrition Information (per serving, serves 4):

- Calories: 110
- Protein: 6g
- Carbohydrates: 2g
- Fat: 9g
- Fiber: 1g
- Sugar: 0g
- Portion Size: 4 skewers

Kale Chips

Ingredients:

- 1 bunch kale, stems removed and leaves torn
- 1 tbsp olive oil
- 1/2 tsp salt

Instructions:

1. Preheat oven to 350°F (175°C).
2. Toss kale with olive oil and salt.
3. Spread on a baking sheet and bake for 10-15 minutes, until crispy.

Nutrition Information (per serving, serves 4):

- Calories: 50

- Protein: 2g
- Carbohydrates: 7g
- Fat: 2g
- Fiber: 2g
- Sugar: 0g
- Portion Size: 1 cup

Greek Yogurt Dip with Veggie Sticks

Ingredients:

- 1 cup Greek yogurt
- 1 tbsp olive oil
- 1 tsp lemon juice
- 1 clove garlic, minced
- Salt and pepper to taste
- Assorted veggie sticks (carrots, bell peppers, celery)

Instructions:

1. Mix yogurt, olive oil, lemon juice, and garlic.
2. Season with salt and pepper.
3. Serve with veggie sticks.

Nutrition Information (per serving, serves 4):

- Calories: 100

- Protein: 5g

- Carbohydrates: 8g

- Fat: 5g

- Fiber: 2g

- Sugar: 4g

- Portion Size: 1/4 cup dip with assorted veggies

Almond Butter Stuffed Celery

Ingredients:

- 4 celery stalks, cut into pieces

- 1/4 cup almond butter

Instructions:

1. Fill celery sticks with almond butter.

Nutrition Information (per serving, serves 4):

- Calories: 90

- Protein: 3g

- Carbohydrates: 6g

- Fat: 7g

- Fiber: 3g

- Sugar: 2g

- Portion Size: 4 pieces

Marinated Artichoke Hearts

Ingredients:

- 1 can artichoke hearts, drained
- 1/4 cup olive oil
- 1/4 cup white wine vinegar
- 1 clove garlic, minced
- 1 tsp dried oregano
- Salt and pepper to taste

Instructions:

1. Mix olive oil, vinegar, garlic, oregano, salt, and pepper.
2. Pour over artichokes and marinate for at least 1 hour.

Nutrition Information (per serving, serves 4):

- Calories: 120
- Protein: 2g
- Carbohydrates: 5g
- Fat: 10g
- Fiber: 2g
- Sugar: 1g
- Portion Size: 1/2 cup

Low Carb Hummus with Bell Pepper Strips

Ingredients:

- 1 can chickpeas, drained and rinsed
- 1/4 cup tahini
- 1/4 cup olive oil
- 1 lemon, juiced
- 1 clove garlic
- Salt to taste
- Bell peppers, cut into strips

Instructions:

1. Blend chickpeas, tahini, olive oil, lemon juice, garlic, and salt until smooth.
2. Serve with bell pepper strips.

Nutrition Information (per serving, serves 4):

- Calories: 160
- Protein: 5g
- Carbohydrates: 13g
- Fat: 10g
- Fiber: 4g
- Sugar: 2g
- Portion Size: 1/4 cup hummus with bell peppers

Mozzarella and Cherry Tomato Skewers

Ingredients:

- 1 cup cherry tomatoes
- 1 cup mozzarella balls
- Fresh basil leaves
- Balsamic glaze for drizzling

Instructions:

1. Thread tomatoes, mozzarella, and basil onto skewers.
2. Drizzle with balsamic glaze.

Nutrition Information (per serving, serves 4):

- Calories: 100
- Protein: 6g
- Carbohydrates: 3g
- Fat: 7g
- Fiber: 1g
- Sugar: 2g
- Portion Size: 4 skewers

Spinach and Artichoke Dip

Ingredients:

- 1 cup frozen spinach, thawed and drained

- 1 can artichoke hearts, drained and chopped
- 1 cup Greek yogurt
- 1/2 cup grated Parmesan cheese
- 1 clove garlic, minced
- Salt and pepper to taste

Instructions:

1. Mix all ingredients in a bowl.
2. Serve chilled or warmed.

Nutrition Information (per serving, serves 4):

- Calories: 120
- Protein: 9g
- Carbohydrates: 7g
- Fat: 6g
- Fiber: 2g
- Sugar: 2g
- Portion Size: 1/2 cup

Zucchini Fritters

Ingredients:

- 2 medium zucchinis, grated
- 1/4 cup almond flour

- 1 egg, beaten
- 1 clove garlic, minced
- Salt and pepper to taste
- Olive oil for frying

Instructions:

1. Mix zucchini, almond flour, egg, garlic, salt, and pepper.
2. Form into small patties.
3. Fry in olive oil until golden brown.

Nutrition Information (per serving, serves 4):

- Calories: 90
- Protein: 3g
- Carbohydrates: 6g
- Fat: 6g
- Fiber: 2g
- Sugar: 2g
- Portion Size: 3 fritters

Caprese Salad Bites

Ingredients:

- 1 cup cherry tomatoes
- 1 cup mozzarella balls

- Fresh basil leaves
- Balsamic glaze for drizzling

Instructions:

1. Thread tomatoes, mozzarella, and basil onto skewers.
2. Drizzle with balsamic glaze.

Nutrition Information (per serving, serves 4):

- Calories: 100
- Protein: 6g
- Carbohydrates: 3g
- Fat: 7g
- Fiber: 1g
- Sugar: 2g
- Portion Size: 4 skewers

Chapter 6: Desserts

When managing Type 2 diabetes, indulging in desserts can be challenging due to the high sugar content typically found in sweet treats. However, with careful planning and the right ingredients, you can enjoy delicious, low-carb desserts that won't spike your blood sugar levels.

Chocolate Avocado Mousse

Ingredients:

- 2 ripe avocados
- 1/4 cup unsweetened cocoa powder
- 1/4 cup almond milk
- 2-3 tablespoons erythritol (or other sugar substitute)
- 1 teaspoon vanilla extract
- Pinch of salt

Instructions:

1. Blend avocados, cocoa powder, almond milk, erythritol, vanilla extract, and salt until smooth.
2. Chill for at least 30 minutes before serving.

Nutrition Information (per serving):

- Calories: 200
- Protein: 3g
- Carbohydrates: 10g
- Fat: 18g
- Fiber: 7g
- Sugar: 1g
- Portion Size: 1/2 cup

Almond Flour Brownies

Ingredients:

- 1 cup almond flour
- 1/2 cup unsweetened cocoa powder
- 1/2 cup erythritol
- 1/2 cup melted coconut oil
- 3 eggs
- 1 teaspoon vanilla extract
- 1/2 teaspoon baking powder
- Pinch of salt

Instructions:

1. Preheat the oven to 350°F (175°C). Grease an 8x8 inch baking pan.

2. Mix all ingredients in a bowl until well combined.

3. Pour the batter into the prepared pan and bake for 20-25 minutes.

4. Let cool before cutting into squares.

Nutrition Information (per serving):

- Calories: 150
- Protein: 4g
- Carbohydrates: 6g
- Fat: 12g
- Fiber: 3g
- Sugar: 1g
- Portion Size: 1 square (1/12 of the pan)

Berry Cheesecake Cups

Ingredients:

- 1 cup mixed berries
- 8 oz cream cheese, softened
- 1/4 cup erythritol
- 1 teaspoon vanilla extract
- 1/2 cup heavy cream

Instructions:

1. Blend cream cheese, erythritol, and vanilla until smooth.

2. Whip the heavy cream until stiff peaks form and fold into the cream cheese mixture.

3. Layer the cheesecake mixture and berries into serving cups.

4. Chill for at least 2 hours before serving.

Nutrition Information (per serving):

- Calories: 250
- Protein: 3g
- Carbohydrates: 8g
- Fat: 22g
- Fiber: 2g
- Sugar: 4g
- Portion Size: 1 cup

Coconut Flour Cookies

Ingredients:

- 1/4 cup coconut flour
- 1/4 cup melted coconut oil
- 1/4 cup erythritol
- 1 egg
- 1 teaspoon vanilla extract

- Pinch of salt

Instructions:

1. Preheat the oven to 350°F (175°C). Line a baking sheet with parchment paper.
2. Mix all ingredients until well combined.
3. Drop spoonfuls of dough onto the prepared baking sheet.
4. Bake for 10-12 minutes, until golden brown.

Nutrition Information (per serving):

- Calories: 90
- Protein: 2g
- Carbohydrates: 4g
- Fat: 8g
- Fiber: 2g
- Sugar: 1g
- Portion Size: 1 cookie

Keto Chocolate Chip Cookies

Ingredients:

- 1 1/2 cups almond flour
- 1/2 cup erythritol
- 1/4 cup melted butter

- 1 egg
- 1/2 teaspoon vanilla extract
- 1/2 teaspoon baking powder
- 1/2 cup sugar-free chocolate chips

Instructions:

1. Preheat the oven to 350°F (175°C). Line a baking sheet with parchment paper.
2. Mix almond flour, erythritol, melted butter, egg, vanilla, and baking powder until combined.
3. Stir in the chocolate chips.
4. Drop spoonfuls of dough onto the prepared baking sheet.
5. Bake for 10-12 minutes, until edges are golden.

Nutrition Information (per serving):

- Calories: 120
- Protein: 3g
- Carbohydrates: 6g
- Fat: 10g
- Fiber: 2g
- Sugar: 1g
- Portion Size: 1 cookie

Lemon Ricotta Cake

Ingredients:

- 1 1/2 cups almond flour
- 1/2 cup erythritol
- 3 eggs
- 1 cup ricotta cheese
- 1/4 cup lemon juice
- Zest of 1 lemon
- 1 teaspoon baking powder
- Pinch of salt

Instructions:

1. Preheat the oven to 350°F (175°C). Grease a 9-inch springform pan.
2. Mix almond flour, erythritol, eggs, ricotta, lemon juice, lemon zest, baking powder, and salt until smooth.
3. Pour batter into the prepared pan.
4. Bake for 35-40 minutes, until a toothpick comes out clean.

Nutrition Information (per serving):

- Calories: 180
- Protein: 6g
- Carbohydrates: 7g
- Fat: 14g

- Fiber: 2g

- Sugar: 2g

- Portion Size: 1 slice (1/8 of the cake)

Chia Seed Pudding with Cocoa

Ingredients:

- 1/4 cup chia seeds

- 1 cup unsweetened almond milk

- 2 tablespoons unsweetened cocoa powder

- 2 tablespoons erythritol

- 1 teaspoon vanilla extract

Instructions:

1. Mix all ingredients in a bowl or jar.

2. Refrigerate for at least 4 hours or overnight, stirring occasionally.

Nutrition Information (per serving):

- Calories: 150

- Protein: 4g

- Carbohydrates: 12g

- Fat: 8g

- Fiber: 9g

- Sugar: 1g
- Portion Size: 1/2 cup

Almond Butter Fat Bombs

Ingredients:

- 1/2 cup almond butter
- 1/4 cup coconut oil
- 2 tablespoons erythritol
- 1 teaspoon vanilla extract
- Pinch of salt

Instructions:

1. Melt almond butter and coconut oil together.
2. Stir in erythritol, vanilla, and salt.
3. Pour into silicone molds and freeze until solid.

Nutrition Information (per serving):

- Calories: 100
- Protein: 2g
- Carbohydrates: 3g
- Fat: 9g
- Fiber: 1g
- Sugar: 1g

- Portion Size: 1 fat bomb

Low Carb Tiramisu

Ingredients:

- 1/2 cup almond flour
- 1/4 cup erythritol
- 1/4 cup melted butter
- 8 oz mascarpone cheese
- 1/2 cup heavy cream
- 1/4 cup strong brewed coffee
- 1 tablespoon unsweetened cocoa powder

Instructions:

1. Mix almond flour, erythritol, and melted butter. Press into the bottom of serving cups.
2. Blend mascarpone and heavy cream until smooth.
3. Layer mascarpone mixture over the crust, drizzle with coffee, and dust with cocoa powder.
4. Chill for at least 2 hours before serving.

Nutrition Information (per serving):

- Calories: 300
- Protein: 4g

- Carbohydrates: 8g
- Fat: 28g
- Fiber: 2g
- Sugar: 1g
- Portion Size: 1 cup

Raspberry Almond Tart

Ingredients:

- 1 cup almond flour
- 1/4 cup melted butter
- 1/4 cup erythritol
- 1/2 cup raspberries
- 1/4 cup sliced almonds

Instructions:

1. Preheat the oven to 350°F (175°C). Grease a tart pan.
2. Mix almond flour, melted butter, and erythritol. Press into the bottom of the pan.
3. Top with raspberries and sliced almonds.
4. Bake for 20-25 minutes.

Nutrition Information (per serving):

- Calories: 180

- Protein: 4g
- Carbohydrates: 6g
- Fat: 16g
- Fiber: 3g
- Sugar: 2g
- Portion Size: 1 slice (1/8 of the tart)

Peanut Butter Chocolate Bars

Ingredients:

- 1 cup natural peanut butter (unsweetened)
- 1/4 cup coconut oil
- 1/4 cup unsweetened cocoa powder
- 2 tablespoons erythritol or stevia
- 1 teaspoon vanilla extract
- Pinch of salt

Instructions:

1. In a microwave-safe bowl, combine peanut butter and coconut oil. Microwave for 30 seconds or until melted.
2. Stir in cocoa powder, erythritol, vanilla extract, and salt until smooth.
3. Pour the mixture into a lined baking dish and refrigerate for 1 hour or until firm.

4. Cut into bars and store in the refrigerator.

Nutrition Information (per serving):

- Calories: 150
- Protein: 4g
- Carbohydrates: 6g
- Fat: 14g
- Fiber: 2g
- Sugar: 1g
- Portion size: 1 bar (makes 10 bars)

Coconut Macaroons

Ingredients:

- 2 cups unsweetened shredded coconut
- 1/4 cup almond flour
- 1/2 cup erythritol or monk fruit sweetener
- 3 egg whites
- 1 teaspoon vanilla extract
- Pinch of salt

Instructions:

1. Preheat the oven to 350°F (175°C). Line a baking sheet with parchment paper.

2. In a large bowl, mix the shredded coconut, almond flour, and sweetener.

3. In a separate bowl, beat the egg whites until stiff peaks form.

4. Fold the egg whites into the coconut mixture along with vanilla extract and salt.

5. Drop spoonfuls of the mixture onto the baking sheet.

6. Bake for 15-20 minutes or until golden brown.

Nutrition Information (per serving):

- Calories: 70
- Protein: 1g
- Carbohydrates: 3g
- Fat: 6g
- Fiber: 2g
- Sugar: 0g
- Portion size: 1 macaroon (makes 20 macaroons)

Sugar-Free Lemon Bars

Ingredients:

For the crust:

- 1 cup almond flour
- 1/4 cup coconut flour
- 1/4 cup melted butter

- 2 tablespoons erythritol

For the filling:

- 3 large eggs
- 1/2 cup lemon juice
- 1/4 cup erythritol
- 2 tablespoons coconut flour

Instructions:

1. Preheat the oven to 350°F (175°C). Line an 8x8-inch baking dish with parchment paper.
2. Mix almond flour, coconut flour, melted butter, and erythritol for the crust. Press into the baking dish and bake for 10 minutes.
3. In a bowl, whisk together eggs, lemon juice, erythritol, and coconut flour for the filling. Pour over the baked crust.
4. Bake for an additional 20 minutes or until the filling is set.
5. Allow to cool before cutting into squares.

Nutrition Information (per serving):

- Calories: 90
- Protein: 3g
- Carbohydrates: 5g
- Fat: 7g

- Fiber: 2g

- Sugar: 0g

- Portion size: 1 bar (makes 16 bars)

Chocolate Chia Pudding

Ingredients:

- 1/4 cup chia seeds

- 1 cup unsweetened almond milk

- 2 tablespoons unsweetened cocoa powder

- 2 tablespoons erythritol or stevia

- 1 teaspoon vanilla extract

Instructions:

1. In a bowl, whisk together chia seeds, almond milk, cocoa powder, sweetener, and vanilla extract.

2. Let the mixture sit for 5 minutes, then stir again to prevent clumping.

3. Cover and refrigerate for at least 1 hour or until thickened.

4. Stir well before serving.

Nutrition Information (per serving):

- Calories: 120

- Protein: 4g

- Carbohydrates: 10g

- Fat: 7g

- Fiber: 7g

- Sugar: 0g

- Portion size: 1/2 cup (makes 4 servings)

Strawberry Cream Cheese Bites

Ingredients:

- 1 cup fresh strawberries, halved

- 4 ounces cream cheese, softened

- 1 tablespoon erythritol or stevia

- 1 teaspoon vanilla extract

Instructions:

1. In a bowl, mix cream cheese, sweetener, and vanilla extract until smooth.
2. Spoon the cream cheese mixture onto each strawberry half.
3. Chill in the refrigerator for 15 minutes before serving.

Nutrition Information (per serving):

- Calories: 50

- Protein: 1g

- Carbohydrates: 3g

- Fat: 4g

- Fiber: 1g

- Sugar: 1g

- Portion size: 2 halves (makes 16 servings)

Chapter 7: Smoothies

Smoothies are an excellent way to incorporate nutrient-dense foods into your diet, especially when managing Type 2 diabetes. They can be quick, delicious, and packed with vitamins, minerals, and fiber, while also being low in carbohydrates.

Green Detox Smoothie

Ingredients:

- 1 cup spinach
- 1/2 cup cucumber
- 1/2 green apple
- 1/2 avocado
- 1 tbsp lemon juice
- 1 cup unsweetened almond milk
- 1 tsp chia seeds

Instructions:

1. Combine all ingredients in a blender.
2. Blend until smooth.
3. Serve immediately.

Nutrition Information (per serving):

- Calories: 180
- Protein: 4g
- Carbohydrates: 15g
- Fat: 12g
- Fiber: 7g
- Sugar: 5g
- Portion Size: 1 serving

Berry Protein Smoothie

Ingredients:

- 1/2 cup mixed berries (strawberries, blueberries, raspberries)
- 1 scoop vanilla protein powder
- 1 cup unsweetened almond milk
- 1 tbsp chia seeds
- 1/2 tsp vanilla extract

Instructions:

1. Place all ingredients in a blender.
2. Blend until smooth.
3. Pour into a glass and enjoy.

Nutrition Information (per serving):

- Calories: 210
- Protein: 20g
- Carbohydrates: 18g
- Fat: 7g
- Fiber: 8g
- Sugar: 10g
- Portion Size: 1 serving

Avocado Spinach Smoothie

Ingredients:

- 1/2 avocado
- 1 cup spinach
- 1/2 banana
- 1 tbsp flaxseeds
- 1 cup coconut water

Instructions:

1. Add all ingredients to a blender.
2. Blend until creamy and smooth.
3. Serve chilled.

Nutrition Information (per serving):

- Calories: 240
- Protein: 3g
- Carbohydrates: 20g
- Fat: 17g
- Fiber: 9g
- Sugar: 7g
- Portion Size: 1 serving

Almond Butter and Banana Smoothie

Ingredients:

- 1 tbsp almond butter
- 1/2 banana
- 1 cup unsweetened almond milk
- 1 tbsp hemp seeds
- 1/2 tsp cinnamon

Instructions:

1. Blend all ingredients until smooth.
2. Pour into a glass and serve.

Nutrition Information (per serving):

- Calories: 230

- Protein: 6g

- Carbohydrates: 22g

- Fat: 14g

- Fiber: 5g

- Sugar: 10g

- Portion Size: 1 serving

Coconut Matcha Smoothie

Ingredients:

- 1 tsp matcha powder

- 1 cup coconut milk

- 1/2 banana

- 1 tbsp shredded coconut

- 1 tsp honey (optional)

Instructions:

1. Combine all ingredients in a blender.

2. Blend until smooth.

3. Enjoy immediately.

Nutrition Information (per serving):

- Calories: 200

- Protein: 2g

- Carbohydrates: 21g

- Fat: 14g

- Fiber: 4g

- Sugar: 10g

- Portion Size: 1 serving

Chocolate Peanut Butter Smoothie

Ingredients:

- 1 tbsp natural peanut butter

- 1 tbsp cocoa powder

- 1/2 banana

- 1 cup unsweetened almond milk

- 1 scoop chocolate protein powder

Instructions:

1. Blend all ingredients until smooth.

2. Serve in a tall glass.

Nutrition Information (per serving):

- Calories: 290

- Protein: 20g

- Carbohydrates: 20g

- Fat: 16g

- Fiber: 6g
- Sugar: 10g
- Portion Size: 1 serving

Kale and Pineapple Smoothie

Ingredients:

- 1 cup kale
- 1/2 cup pineapple chunks
- 1/2 banana
- 1 cup coconut water
- 1 tbsp chia seeds

Instructions:

1. Place all ingredients in a blender.
2. Blend until smooth and creamy.
3. Serve immediately.

Nutrition Information (per serving):

- Calories: 180
- Protein: 3g
- Carbohydrates: 30g
- Fat: 5g
- Fiber: 7g

- Sugar: 17g
- Portion Size: 1 serving

Blueberry Almond Smoothie

Ingredients:

- 1/2 cup blueberries
- 1 tbsp almond butter
- 1 cup unsweetened almond milk
- 1 tbsp flaxseed meal
- 1/2 tsp vanilla extract

Instructions:

1. Add all ingredients to the blender.
2. Blend until smooth.
3. Enjoy cold.

Nutrition Information (per serving):

- Calories: 190
- Protein: 4g
- Carbohydrates: 18g
- Fat: 12g
- Fiber: 6g
- Sugar: 10g

- Portion Size: 1 serving

Spinach and Mint Smoothie

Ingredients:

- 1 cup spinach
- 1/4 cup fresh mint leaves
- 1/2 cucumber
- 1/2 green apple
- 1 cup unsweetened almond milk

Instructions:

1. Combine all ingredients in a blender.
2. Blend until smooth and well combined.
3. Serve immediately.

Nutrition Information (per serving):

- Calories: 110
- Protein: 3g
- Carbohydrates: 16g
- Fat: 4g
- Fiber: 4g
- Sugar: 8g
- Portion Size: 1 serving

Pumpkin Pie Smoothie

Ingredients:

- 1/2 cup pumpkin puree
- 1/2 banana
- 1 cup unsweetened almond milk
- 1/2 tsp pumpkin pie spice
- 1 tbsp chia seeds

Instructions:

1. Blend all ingredients until smooth.
2. Pour into a glass and enjoy.

Nutrition Information (per serving):

- Calories: 150
- Protein: 3g
- Carbohydrates: 25g
- Fat: 5g
- Fiber: 6g
- Sugar: 10g
- Portion Size: 1 serving

Strawberry Kiwi Smoothie

Ingredients:

- 1/2 cup strawberries
- 1 kiwi, peeled
- 1 cup unsweetened coconut water
- 1 tbsp chia seeds
- 1/2 banana

Instructions:

1. Place all ingredients in a blender.
2. Blend until smooth.
3. Serve immediately.

Nutrition Information (per serving):

- Calories: 140
- Protein: 2g
- Carbohydrates: 31g
- Fat: 2g
- Fiber: 7g
- Sugar: 18g
- Portion Size: 1 serving

Vanilla Chai Smoothie

Ingredients:

- 1 cup unsweetened almond milk
- 1/2 frozen banana
- 1/2 tsp vanilla extract
- 1/2 tsp chai spice blend
- 1 scoop vanilla protein powder

Instructions:

1. Add all ingredients to the blender.
2. Blend until smooth and creamy.
3. Serve immediately.

Nutrition Information (per serving):

- Calories: 210
- Protein: 22g
- Carbohydrates: 19g
- Fat: 6g
- Fiber: 4g
- Sugar: 10g
- Portion Size: 1 serving

Raspberry Coconut Smoothie

Ingredients:

- 1/2 cup raspberries
- 1/2 cup coconut milk
- 1/2 banana
- 1 tbsp chia seeds
- 1/2 tsp vanilla extract

Instructions:

1. Combine all ingredients in a blender.
2. Blend until smooth.
3. Pour into a glass and enjoy.

Nutrition Information (per serving):

- Calories: 180
- Protein: 2g
- Carbohydrates: 20g
- Fat: 11g
- Fiber: 6g
- Sugar: 10g
- Portion Size: 1 serving

Mango and Coconut Smoothie

Ingredients:

- 1/2 cup mango chunks
- 1/2 cup coconut milk
- 1/2 banana
- 1 tbsp flaxseeds
- 1/2 cup ice

Instructions:

1. Place all ingredients in a blender.
2. Blend until smooth and creamy.
3. Serve chilled.

Nutrition Information (per serving):

- Calories: 170
- Protein: 2g
- Carbohydrates: 25g
- Fat: 8g
- Fiber: 4g
- Sugar: 18g
- Portion Size: 1 serving

Lemon Ginger Smoothie

Ingredients:

- 1/2 lemon, juiced
- 1/2 inch ginger root
- 1/2 banana
- 1 cup unsweetened almond milk
- 1 tbsp chia seeds

Instructions:

1. Add all ingredients to a blender.
2. Blend until smooth.
3. Pour into a glass and enjoy.

Nutrition Information (per serving):

- Calories: 130
- Protein: 3g
- Carbohydrates: 22g
- Fat: 4g
- Fiber: 5g
- Sugar: 10g
- Portion Size: 1 serving

CONCLUSION

As we reach the end of "Low Carb Vegetarian Meal Plan for Type 2 Diabetes," it's essential to reflect on the journey we have embarked upon together. This book has been designed to provide you with the tools, knowledge, and inspiration necessary to manage Type 2 diabetes through a healthy, low carb, vegetarian diet. By following the carefully crafted meal plans and diverse recipes, you have taken a significant step towards improving your health and overall well-being.

Throughout the chapters, we've explored a wide array of delicious and nutritious recipes that demonstrate how varied and enjoyable a low carb vegetarian diet can be. From hearty breakfasts to satisfying dinners, tasty snacks, indulgent desserts, and refreshing smoothies, this book ensures that every meal can be both diabetes-friendly and flavorful.

The subsequent chapters offered a treasure trove of recipes, each designed to be low in carbohydrates yet rich in nutrients. By incorporating a variety of vegetables, plant-based proteins, healthy fats, and whole foods, these recipes help stabilize blood sugar levels, promote weight management, and enhance overall health.

As you continue on this path, remember that consistency is key. The tips and strategies provided in the conclusion will support you in maintaining this lifestyle long-term. Celebrate your progress, no matter how small, and stay motivated by the improvements in your health and vitality.

This book is more than just a collection of recipes; it's a roadmap to a healthier, more vibrant life. Embrace the variety of flavors, experiment with new ingredients, and find joy in preparing meals that nourish your body and mind.

Your journey doesn't end here. Keep exploring, learning, and adapting as needed. Utilize the resources and further reading suggestions to deepen your understanding and stay inspired. Most importantly, remember that you are not alone. There is a community of individuals on similar journeys, and together, we can support each other in achieving our health goals.

Thank you for allowing this book to be a part of your journey. Here's to your health, happiness, and a future filled with delicious, diabetes-friendly meals.